Say Yes more often.

---

Risk + failure = growth

---

Find time for your child today.

---

Time together is never a waste.

---

Model the behavior that we want.

---

Consistency, Consistency,

Consistency

---

Anger is just a self-protective device.

---

Look at struggles as areas of opportunity.

---

Give your child time and love, not things.

---

Children demand time, not parenting skills.

---

Care enough for your kids to set boundaries.

---

Your time is all that children really

want.

---

Failure with Praise = Risk & Risk over time = Growth

---

kid's who know how to lose get way ahead in life.

---

Love your spouse more than you love your children.

---

Marriage is permanent while parenthood is passing.

---

We all like to laugh - we should do it more often.

---

Never give up. I've tried everything is not a good answer.

---

Do not assume you know what your teen is thinking.

---

We often pay a great price for trying to be perfect.

---

Don't sacrifice the relationship for the rules.

---

Pick your battles! Not everything is a major offense.

Angry teens are simply telling you that they are sad.

---

Winning at work doesn't mean much if we fail at life.

---

Law of Indispensability. Only do

what only you can do.

---

Discipline isn't about punishment it is about learning.

---

We need to be clear even when we might not feel certain.

---

There is always hope for your teen if you never give up.

---

do not take more control than you need to keep them safe.

---

Be sure to say, I am sorry, I made a mistake.

Embrace every stage and phase of childhood development.

---

Don't try to prove your parenting skill by doing everything.

The less you do, the more you enable your kids to accomplish.

---

Bless your kids with all the disadvantages required for success.

---

Laugh at yourself and build your identity beyond that of parent.

---

Memories are always filled with stories of time spent together.

---

Time is the ultimate gift. Shower your child with this blessing.

---

If you fight in front of the kids, let

them also see you make up.

---

The secret of concentration is elimination. Dr. Howard Hendricks

---

Ask open-ended questions that require more than one-word responses.

---

A gentle response diffuses anger. Practice using a softer voice.

---

Calm yourself down. Teens don't hear us when we are out of control.

---

Be sure to say, I'm sorry, I made a

mistake.

---

Once words are out, you cannot take them back. Control your tongue.

---

Anger can destroy the teaching opportunity that discipline provides.

---

Act like the leader of the home. Be authentic and straightforward.

---

Timing is everything when there are important issues to be discussed.

---

Mostly, what teens need from

parents is to simply be there for them.

---

Make sure your kids see you showing physical affection to your spouse.

---

Leadership in the home or in the office starts with being self-aware.

It is ok and actually important to parent different kids differently.

---

Be spontaneous - drop everything and do something way out of character.

---

Anger directed at your teen will heighten their resolve for opposition.

---

Practice what you preach because parenting is caught, not simply taught.

---

Use humor to diffuse tense situations without making light of the issue.

---

Take a time out and show your child how to take a breathe and calm down.

---

Parenting requires courage. Success

can only happen when we move forward.

---

Don't dwarf your child's personality by being too possessive as a parent.

---

Tell your children about the lessons they have taught you over the years.

---

Self worth is the result of feeling valued and loved just for who you are.

---

Parent your kids according to their personality not a formula or tradition.

Nothing paralyzes our lives like the attitude that things can never change.

---

It is difficult to find a delinquent teen that comes from a harmonious home.

Ask your kids their opinions about things that are totally unrelated to them.

---

Parents that demonstrate healthy love see mistakes as opportunities to learn.

---

Note to self: It's all about the relationship, stupid.

---

Challenge your teen and stimulate discussion but always with positive support.

---

Rules in the home function as a map for kids to navigate through to adulthood.

---

Do birthdays big! Money is not necessary to make the day all about your child.

---

Try to conquer life's struggles one at a time. Too many goals clouds progress.

Over protection sends an implied message, I do not believe you are capable.

---

A home without rules is like trying to build a tower of blocks on a trampoline.

Your attitude toward yourself as a parent will affect your child's self esteem.

---

do not take responsibility for things that your teen should do for themselves.

---

Give your child an opportunity to make a choice today and live with the results.

---

Try to interpret depression and anger as confusion and not as a personal insult.

---

You can be a parent without character, but you won't be a leader worth following.

---

Loving relationships with our children require a commitment of time and effort.

---

Do not be afraid to be disliked by

your children when you're enforcing the rules.

---

Time is valuable. Make sure you are using it on the things you really care about.

---

Perception is everything. Kids respond to their interpretation, not to the truth.

---

Arguments are counterproductive and resistance is a signal to change strategies.

---

Providing clear restrictions for kids helps them navigate their complicated world.

Start and maintain some unique family traditions that only your family knows about.

---

When we feel out of control as parents, we tend to over control those around us.

Even hostile angry teens are extremely sensitive to the feeling of not being loved.

Angry teens are trying to gain attention and increase care, not distance themselves.

Do less, accomplish more. Become more competent through reflection and concentration.

---

Randomly text your kids some encouraging words. It shows you're thinking about them.

---

*Willingness to say no to opportunities is often what sets leader apart from the pack.*

---

*Look what you might need to change about yourself before you find fault in your kids.*

---

*When you inject humor into the*

home it can remove a mountain of relational tension.

---

Find ways to slow down your anger through exercise, relaxation, or taking a time-out.

---

Adversity is your opportunity to deepen your commitment and

connection to loved ones.

---

Inappropriate behavior is a quick way to gain significance in the adolescent economy.

---

Become an observer of your thoughts as opposed to being a prisoner to your thoughts.

---

*Meaningful, lasting change in our lives requires three things: time, grace and truth.*

---

*Get down to your child's physical level when talking to them. Face to face is critical.*

Kids crave intensity whether positive or negative. Be careful what you're intense about.

It is better to be on the wrong page with your spouse than on the right page by yourself.

The rapid body growth of teen's during adolescence requires at least nine hours of sleep.

---

Healthy love means nurturing our kids to be unique and not focusing on them being perfect.

---

*It is generally impossible to get teens to do what you want them to do by talking to them.*

---

*Teens often operate out of impulse and do not respect parents that are paralyzed by fear.*

---

*We live in an age of anxiety.*

Confidence is an important gift to pass along to your child.

---

Communicate in a way that makes it easy for your teen to understand your intended subject.

---

You know you are overindulging your child if you only consider their interests and needs.

---

Discern what lies your child believes about him or herself and speak truth to their hearts.

---

Minimize the risk of cyberbullying by keeping the computer in a busy location of the house.

---

Spend time with your child so that you have the best possible chance of knowing your child.

---

The slow speed of your teen is not an insult directed at you so do not take it personally.

---

Everyone has insecurities. Humanize your approach to parenting by admitting your own fears.

---

Teens that exhibit depression or anger need more communication with their parents, not less.

Do you speak to your partner or teen in a way that allows them to understand your feelings?

---

Issues of character and the heart are more important than issues of behavior. Be discerning.

Let your teen shave off/color their hair if they want to. It is only hair; it will grow back.

---

Eat at least 3-4 meals a week together. Sit around afterward and just relax with each other.

---

Stop protecting your child and give them a chance to manage something that seems beyond them.

---

Tell your children what lessons you have learned from them and what traits you admire in them.

---

Over possessive and over permissive

parents build insecurity into the lives of their children.

---

Perfectionists often strive after higher values, even at the cost of great personal sacrifice.

---

Half of parenting is what you do not do and what you do not allow yourself to get dragged into.

---

Time defines value. If you don't give it to your kids they will assume that their value is low.

---

Good habits are the key to school performance. Help your child develop the process of learning.

---

Cheer for mistakes and loses. This will expand your child's willingness to take risks and grow.

---

Find a mentor. No matter how impressive your skills might be, coaching always improves outcomes.

---

You might be overprotecting your child if you see them as fragile and do not allow for mistakes.

---

Do you take responsibility for how your teen is feeling? You can't rescue them from everything.

---

Anger and depression feel intimidating and challenging, but they are really just a cry for help.

---

Don't be the parent that is afraid to let your child fail. Allow failure to teach and strengthen.

---

As a parent, you should only do in the home what only you can do. Allow your kids to do the rest.

---

Do not believe the myth that everything we say or do as parents will have an everlasting effect.

---

What are some things you might

trust your child with to surprise them and build their confidence?

---

Convince yourself that your teen does want to talk to you even though he/she might not admit it.

---

Make the most of the car rides. Use this one-on-one time to really listen, connect and encourage.

---

Children push against rules not in an effort to break through, but to ensure that they are there.

---

Do not rescue your teen.  The less you do as a parent, the more you enable your teen to accomplish.

---

*Find a way to join your teen in their world. Affirmation through participation is a powerful gift.*

---

*Be mission-driven rather than need-driven. Move through life with purpose rather than with reaction.*

---

Identify your own feelings of anger and use them as a signal of problems that need to be addressed.

---

Too often we bend everything for the child's benefit or wishes. This creates self-centered children.

---

Most conversations that have one's feelings as the subject don't need a clear action plan to follow.

---

Take pictures of the good times to help remind both you and your teen of when things made more sense.

---

Mistakes are a great opportunity for parents to teach so do not miss out by minimizing the behavior.

---

It seems like a no-brainer, but tell your kids you love them every day whether they deserve it or not.

---

Get out of the house and enjoy the outdoors together even if it is just sitting on a playground swing.

---

You can't stop the battle being waged daily for your teens soul, but you can fight on your teens side.

---

In the words of Erma Bombeck:

...normal is just a setting on the dryer... Live in your child's box

---

Stand for something in life. Demonstrate this resolve and strength in your interactions in the home.

---

Provide your child with a sense of

accomplishment and significance by letting them make more decisions.

---

Cyberbullying is most common in middle school. Pay attention to what your kids are experiencing online.

---

Uncertain times within the home

require clear directives. Don't allow uncertainty to leave you paralyzed.

---

You have got to make a lot of deposits into the credibility bank before you can risk making a withdrawal.

---

Anger and emotion are

counterproductive to parenting. Protect your energy by staying calm and objective.

---

Emotions always cloud our ability to reason and develop effective strategies for leadership in the home.

---

Children grow in their own self-confidence when they sense love, trust and loyalty between their parents.

---

If your child is struggling with who they are, reassure them that this is not a permanent state of being.

---

We learn the most from experience. Let go of some of your expectations and simply have fun with your kids.

---

It is not our responsibility to produce change. As parents we are only required to provide opportunities.

---

We need 4 hugs a day for survival. We need 8 hugs a day for maintenance. We need 12 hugs a day for growth.

---

Tell more jokes. You might be surprised how easy it is to draw even hostile kids back into a conversation.

---

Disconnection with our teens happens when we as parents over-control, overprotect, or overindulge our kids.

---

How we disciple conveys our intention. Anger can destroy the teaching opportunity that discipline provides.

---

Enjoy the mundane moments with your children. Just being with your child as significant long lasting value.

---

Be careful how you talk about your kids friends: in their minds, rejecting their friends is rejecting them.

---

Boundaries are critical to kids of all ages because they help the child determine their path into adulthood.

---

Ask yourself, What is my responsibility and objective? Have a purpose and a plan when parenting.

---

Have - no technology - or - no electricity - nights where you shut everything off and camp in the living room.

---

Be sure your words match your belief. Be sure your teen sees a genuineness and honesty in you as their parent.

---

Let teens complete their sentences. Interrupting makes them feel as if their ideas are not worth listening to.

---

Take 20 seconds and search

through your head and your heart to identify the feelings that are most prevalent.

---

When times are difficult with your teen, crack open a photo album and remember the special gift that they are.

---

Commitment to character might require saying no to what many would perceive to be an opportunity of a lifetime.

---

Parents that overindulge their kids are often kind rather than firm and tend to believe mistakes do not matter.

---

Join Facebook, Twitter and Tumblr and use the technological tools that your children are using. Stay relevant.

---

It is ok if your teen learns that life is not fair and neither are you. Perfection is not an appropriate goal.

---

Do not laugh at your kids when you're not supposed to. Sarcasm kills all relationships and is toxic with kids.

---

Promise to quit faking or exaggerating your anger. Instead, tell the truth and ask directly for what you need.

---

If your teen ignores your requests to verbal conversation, try communicating through email, texting or Facebook.

---

do not fall into the routine of life. Keep it flexible and fun by altering the schedule and your expectations.

---

A bold move as a parent often makes you seem even more powerful in the eyes of your child than you actually are.

---

Focus on the relationship and your child will have all the good feelings that they need to move forward in life.

---

When we over-control, we crush our kids' spirit and hinder their ability to grow into strong, independent adults.

---

Be fun to live with. Teens might be hard to have in the home sometimes, but how easy are you to spend time with?

---

Most teens are unsure of what they feel. So do not expect them to share their lack of insight and understanding.

---

Pass up opportunities to insult,

attack, or criticize. Letting go of your opinion is not as easy as it sounds.

---

Lions circle hesitant prey. Parenting with timidity can be dangerous and hesitation will effect your execution.

---

It isn't consistency that kids crave it is clarity. But clarity becomes more difficult when you are inconsistent.

---

If you enter a parental decision with less than total confidence you will create more obstacles than you'll solve.

---

Bring laughter into the home every day. Embrace the adolescent in your life and have fun with this stage of life.

---

Love for your child should be the result of the love that you share between each other as parents, not instead of.

Start off by saying, I don't need you to agree with me or fix me, I just want you to understand how I am feeling.

---

Teens are so focused on independence and separation that they struggle to admit a need for direction and support.

---

*Taking yourself less seriously will help your child to feel more accepted and free to fully express him or herself.*

---

*Your children are watching you. Everything you do might not be remembered, but it does teach and* will be emulated.

---

Ambivalence about change is normal and can be resolved by working with your teens intrinsic motivations and values.

---

Our kids can really pull on our heartstrings and we should respond promptly to real needs, but not always give in.

---

Be united in front of the kids - deal with your discrepancies in private. Let them see that you support each other.

---

Gifts should be given in an effort to

communicate love, not buy it. Give things that connect to your teen's heart.

---

Teens body language and verbal language do not often match. Take time to understand and do not jump to conclusions.

---

Say less and do more. Give the gift of time and watch your kids share your beliefs without you having to say a word.

---

People who have followed us are exactly where we have led them. Don't blame your teen if they love television.

---

Remember that your children are people too - entitled to their own way of doing things, and their own way of thinking.

---

Encouragement is great, but giving undeserved or excessive praise weakens your ability to motivate and challenge them.

---

Over-controlling parents give directions and commands. Healthy parental love practices collaborative problem solving.

---

Monitor your child's digital world. Knowing their passwords is not a violation of privacy - it is healthy supervision.

---

Know your child's online friends as well as their off-line friends. Both groups may be having a significant influence.

---

Make a family bucket list and commit to doing one or two things on the list every year, even after they leave the home.

---

Don't assume that your kids hate to do things that you hate to do. Allow your kids to show some of their unique skills.

---

Remember that the brain is not fully developed until we are 25 years old. Do not expect your teen to speak with logic.

---

Always say less than necessary. Do not make it easy for an emotional teen to be side tracked with your extra comments.

---

Too much freedom in the home

creates confusion and a wandering through adolescence that usually ends in disappointment.

---

Pull them out of school and do something special together. Show them that you value them more than what they achieve.

---

The momentary satisfaction you gain through sarcasm will be outweighed by the price you pay through the loss of loyalty.

---

Children require an education in hope. Don't allow the fears of the world to overwhelm the discussions within your home.

---

Encourage the feeling of worth and significance by trusting your child occasionally with things that surprise the child.

---

Help your child perform to their highest ability by knowing them. See the child in front of you. Let go of comparisons.

---

As adults we do not like bosses that are demanding and always sharing their personal critiques. Your kids do not either.

---

Allow your kids to have a say in their consequences. Often they will be harsher on themselves than you were going to be.

---

A child that feels pressured to be superior and excel rather than being themselves, will develop feelings of inferiority.

---

Don't be fooled into thinking that the parent-child relationship should take priority over the husband-wife relationship.

---

Even little children are big enough to give forgiveness when you make a mistake so be sure to ask them for it when needed.

---

Great parenting requires courage and clarity.  Step through feelings of uncertainty with initiative and clear directives.

---

Speak to your teen in a way that gives them a better chance of understanding how you feel instead of just talking at them.

---

Personality develops through making

decisions. Give your child a chance to develop their self worth through decision-making.

---

We want our kids to have toughness and grit but we are afraid of the process that helps them get there. Let your child fail.

---

Find deep connection in at least one relationship so that you can receive honest feedback and support in your parenting role.

---

Develop your total self and enlarge your identity within the home. Lead your teens by showing them rather than telling them.

---

Determine what fuels the rebellious behavior. Move past the surface behavior to find the need that acting out it is filling.

---

If your teen avoids looking at you when telling you a story or looks at you too long without blinking -- he/she may be lying.

---

Teens who feel worthless will often play keep away with the relationships that are actually the most important to them.

---

Anger is a rush and can be addictive. The surge of adrenaline activates the body and can inject excitement into a dull day.

---

When children are the center of attention they look at the world in terms of what they can get instead of what they can give.

---

Nothing but love should come for free. do not shelter your teen from this reality. Let them experience the struggle of life.

---

What do teens most value and admire in a parent? Teens want to see their parents demonstrating integrity and self motivation.

---

Do not be blinded by current difficulties with your child. Look back through photo albums to remind yourself of better times.

---

Be the same person in the home as outside of it lest your family sees you as a hypocrite and you lose influence and authority.

---

Children test boundaries and rules

as a way to determine the level of love and support that their parents are able to provide.

---

Develop interests outside your role as a parent. Take up a hobby, join a health club, or volunteer in the community. Balance

---

When your kids friends come over, put pants on. No really, try to respect their friends no matter how strange they might look.

---

Even if you do not feel love toward your teen a small gift can open the lines of communication and remind us of our connection.

---

Be optimistic and hopeful. Teens are sensitive to pessimism and will not follow someone who lacks faith in their own abilities.

---

Spoiling breeds discontent, but working alongside your teen to help them achieve success builds relationship and responsibility.

---

Keeping your teen off balance by not falling into predictable roles will help expand your identity and keep communication fresh.

---

Self care often begins with building structure into a life with healthy habits. Practice what you preach. Go for a walk today.

---

Develop a sense of adequacy in your child by finding one thing today that you can affirm and encourage in your child's behavior.

---

Entitlement kills. Practice saying no to your kids when they are young or spend a lifetime locked in a battle with selfishness.

---

Find balance in parenting. If you are too uptight than let go and have some fun. Find ways for your kids to express themselves.

---

Small gifts can communicate what words cannot. Do not try to buy love, but practice doing nice things when they aren't expected.

---

See the big picture. do not let the details of life distract you from the relationship you are trying to create with your child.

---

Teens engage in risky behavior for a

purpose. Often it's used to gain a sense of significance that they were missing as children.

---

do it yourself - you will be doing everything for your kids long into adulthood. Give them a chance and prepare them for life.

---

*Write your feelings out before sharing them. You might find that the voices in your head have a harsher message than you intend.*

---

*An emotional response to a situation will cost you a lot more than any temporary satisfaction you get by expressing your feelings.*

---

A sense of inferiority begins early in life. Notice your child when they are young before they force you to notice them as teens.

---

Drug use is often simply a tool to runaway from problems. When a person feels secure and safe, the need to run is greatly reduced.

---

All the good advice in the world isn't going to change the situation with your children at certain times in your relationship.

---

Tell your kids you are proud of who they are, not just what they do. Find the positive aspects of their character and go overboard.

---

Learn the difference between a dilemma, a crisis, and an emergency. Not every difference of opinion should be handled the same way.

---

Do not protect yourself in the heat of teen battles. Open yourself up and watch your teen follow you to a deeper level of sincerity.

---

Figure out your child's personality type and then discuss it with them. They love learning about themselves and what makes them tick.

---

Anger is often used to gain power,

create distance, or avoid real feelings. What are you trying to accomplish when you are losing it?

---

Unexpected gifts can open your child's heart. Simple tokens like a note in their lunch can soften tension and build the relationship.

---

Hug your teen even when you don't feel like it. Our sons and daughters need to sense that we are connecting with them on a heart level.

---

Building your child's self-esteem should not be your primary goal. Self-esteem is a natural outcome of a strong parental relationship.

---

Pursue your kids and express your love daily. If you get to the end of the day and realize you haven't made a connection, go make one.

---

Be your kid's friend on Facebook and make friends with as many of theirs as you can. Use the insight to speak into them.

---

Teens often have a very negative inner dialog so do not add to it by suggesting they are not good enough, do not belong or are unlovable.

---

Kids seem to have a repertoire of hooks they use to get their parents to argue with them. Learn to recognize and avoid these.

---

Spend time with your teen's friends. The better they know you, the less likely they will be to pressure your teen to break family rules.

---

Life provides a limited number of

opportunities for children to build character. Try not to protect them from these natural consequences.

---

A willingness to lose or fail is critical to growth. Be as proud of the losses as the successes and watch your child move forward in life.

---

Instead of a lecture, try an activity. Find ways to connect with your teen that don't involve a lesson but are purely for fun.

---

Do not expect your teen to be good at everything. Help them find where they add unique value to the world and watch their work ethic soar.

---

Do not use morality as a tactic in a fight with your teen. The inferiority they will feel will only build future resentment and hostility.

---

Teens are looking for rules and boundaries as a way to determine their own behavior. They want the support of parents to provide direction.

---

Life has a way of always feeling rushed. Teach your kids how to prioritize in life by slowing down and not trying to accomplish everything.

---

Also, in the words of Erma Bombeck...normal is just a setting on the dryer...live in your child's box, not someone else's.

---

Children's talking, thinking and reasoning are, by definition, immature. They are often inconsistent. Breathe deeply and let some of it go.

---

In order to reach understanding between you and your teen, it will require the two of you to search for the meaning behind the conversation.

---

Moms and dads are more committed to the task of parenting

than ever, but kids often behave in entitled ways. Loving too much can be harmful.

---

Practice taking responsibility for your own life. The more you own, the less time you might have to take responsibility for your teen's life.

---

do not stifle emotional growth because you see your teen's self expression as disrespect or back talk. Stimulate conversation...do not end it.

---

Do not major on minor issues. There are choices that each child makes that are not that big of a deal in the grand scheme of life!

---

*Character provides our kids with the moral compass necessary to attract positive peers and the adult support necessary to move forward in life.*

---

*Time goes by quickly and every stage has its joys and struggles. do not focus on the future so much that* you miss the good things in the present.

---

Fight the urge to jump to conclusions. Because we all were teenagers before, we often assume we know what our teen is trying to express or hide.

---

Affirming words from moms and dads are like switches. Speak a word of affirmation at the right moment and watch even your older children light up.

---

Teens resist leadership through arguing, interrupting, denying, and ignoring. Roll with this resistance and maintain your vision for your family.

---

Let teens speak for themselves. They don't need representation at school, jobs, or in public. Build their self-confidence by trusting their voice.

---

Parents need to develop a different skill set than what they used when their kids were younger. Stay flexible and willing to grow with your child.

---

Parental permissiveness might be in vogue, but it often leaves kids feeling insecure and unable to build their own personality on a firm foundation.

---

Breath slowly and deeply when you approach your teen. It removes the tension from your face and allows the conversation to start from a safer place.

---

Share a donut together. Small treats that are shared have special meaning to kids of all ages. Kids notice when you inconvenience yourself for them.

---

A leader in the home demonstrates initiative and integrity. The character traits that we hope for in our kids need to be modeled by us parents first.

---

Remember that eighty percent of

communication is accomplished through body language. Manage your body more closely when conversations are heating up.

---

Time outs are not just a punishment for children, but an excellent way for parents to reclaim a calm spirit and come back ready to listen more deeply.

---

Parents often feel intimidated by their teen and refrain from asking questions.  do not try to keep them happy by not setting limits or expectations.

---

Parents today tend to give in excessively. Teach you child how to improvise by expecting that they will first try to get their wants met on their own.

---

Teens tend to have an inflated ego. They need this hightened level of confidence if they are going to leave home and try to make it on the their own.

---

*The emotional well-being of a child is affected more by the relationship between the parents than by the direct relationship between parent and child.*

---

*Self-centered children react, rebel or runaway when they don't get what they want. Remove them from the center of your life and order will be restored.*

---

Go puddle jumping. Behave like a kid sometimes and laugh together. Parenting is more than a teaching job - it's okay to have fun and enjoy each other.

---

As parents we often have preconceived ideas about how our

kids should turn out. Let go of this pressure and you and your family will find greater joy.

---

Teens have a desire for power, but they are clumsy in their efforts to gain authority over their own lives. Help them gain power without 'killing' you.

---

Every child is special but every child is not especially good at everything. Encourage your teen to be an expert in somethings but not in everything.

---

It is natural to clamp down on our kids when we are feeling overwhelmed and anxious. Projecting our own insecurities onto our children weighs them down.

---

We all need and want approval, acceptance, and validation from others. If you do not provide these gifts for your teen, they will look for it elsewhere.

---

Maintain a calm attitude by

reminding yourself that you and your teen are actually separate people and that you are not responsible for his/her mistakes.

---

No matter how practiced and skilled, when your teen lies, they will get defensive and grumpy. Check-up on their story and watch the behavior escalate.

---

Venting your anger will often leave you feeling guilty, stupid, and out of control. Find ways to release impatience and frustration before it builds up.

---

As parents we want to give our kids everything we thought we should have had. But we need to hold ourselves back and provided what is needed, not wanted.

---

Mobility might help your career, but it can create instability in the life of your child. Surround your child with love and structure if you need to move.

---

Be mindful of your reputation within the home. You can't expect your teen to manage stress with calmness if you lose your temper when tough stuff happens.

---

We should not use anger so often that it becomes an expected emotion. Anger rarely gets long term results and often hinders future leadership in the home.

---

Don't major on minor issues. There are choices that each child makes that are not that big of a deal in the grand scheme of life!

---

How do you feel when someone disagrees with you? Maybe it is time to work on yourself more than on your kids. Focus on humility, empathy, and flexibility.

---

If you want your teen to listen to you it is critical that you are authentic. Be straightforward; tell your teen what you stand for and then stand for it.

---

*What kind of home environment are you fostering? Would you want to live in your house? Take a step back and try seeing things from your teen's perspective.*

---

*If you want your teen to change his or her behavior, look at yourself. How you interact with your teen has a huge impact in how they think, feel, and behave.*

---

Do a big project together. Build a boat, fix a bike, make a 7-course meal. This not only creates memories, but also provides a platform to interact and talk.

---

Parenting is a great education in understanding people. Teens are brilliant at hiding their motivations in the cloud of dust which surrounds their behaviors.

---

If every disagreement results in your teens losing the battle they will begin to use more powerful techniques to win. Win the war by sacrificing some battles.

---

We can't ask our teens to change unless we have a vision for what we are trying to accomplish. Take some time today to reflect and determine what is important.

---

The goal of parenting is to become unnecessary. Much like with training a new employee, you need to find ways for your teen to practice what they are learning.

---

Distinguish between authority and competency. Share areas of responsibility with family members that might actually be more skilled. Even if you have authority.

---

Overindulging your child creates an

addiction or need for the next best thing. As the newness of the new toy wears off, the cycle of dissatisfaction will set in.

---

Over teaching is like over reaching, you will stumble and fall. Let some teachable moments slip by. You do not need to make parenting one long lecture circuit.

---

Teen rebellion often invokes our own anger. Let go of logic and try to use your heart to speak to your teen. Show love and care even when it might be undeserved.

---

Speak into your child his or her identity. Tell them who they were when they were little and the positive aspects that they have carried with them from childhood.

---

Letting your child struggle is OK. Don't believe the lie that, Good parents do everything they can to keep their children from struggling.

---

Parenting is not a task; it is a

relationship. Stop trying to teach appropriate behavior and start listening because you care and want to learn about who they are.

---

Look for ways to stimulate your kids. Make them think. Keep them on their toes by asking unique questions when their attention is captive at dinner or on a drive.

---

We all assume we are better at more things than we really are. Help your teen learn how to narrow his abilities into excellence rather than expand them into failures.

---

Cultivate an attitude of optimism within the home. If you have lost hope, how do you think your less experienced teen is going to find the confidence to move forward?

---

Refrain from talking poorly about your teen's friends. They identify with their friends and so a negative comment about a friend is a sharp arrow into their own heart.

---

Smart fish do not bite. If your teen is fishing for your anger, turn down the bait. Do not give your teen an opportunity to use your anger and frustration against you.

---

It is imperative for the character development of children that they be allowed to face age-appropriate challenges on their own with the support of loving encouragement.

---

Take your kids on dates: give them a little bit of money to spend on anything they want. No matter their age everyone likes to buy a treat and it will create a memory.

---

The brain is not fully developed until age 25. Expect some bizarre thinking and acting out as the brain builds connections that only time and experience can strengthen.

---

Parental conflict creates tension in the home. Tension leads to insecurity in kids. Kids deal with insecurity by using drugs, cutting themselves or exhibiting hostility.

---

We all want our kids to succeed. Too much parental involvement can backfire and actually hinder growth because the child never learns how to take personal responsibility.

---

Take your role as a parent only as seriously as you absolutely must. Remember why you had kids. It wasn't to be 'boss' in your own house but rather to have a connection.

---

The loss of a spouse or suddenly becoming a single parent can push parents to hold on to their children more closely. The lack of emotional space will hinder their growth.

---

As negative peer pressure threatens to tilt teens towards unhealthy living, tip the scale the other direction by spending time with your teen doing something new and fresh.

---

Find ways to relate to your kids that will enhance your authority as a parent and increase your effectiveness. Try going for a walk and focusing on their story and struggle.

---

Some parents are so fearful of pressures teens face that they try to shield their kids from the influence of their peers. Let them get battle ready in age appropriate ways.

---

*Somehow we seem to be tough in our work world but fail to bring this same resolve and energy into the home. Demonstrate passion in the home and find your purpose as a parent.*

---

*Our kids started sleeping through the night when we started wearing* ear plugs. Sometimes the best intervention is 'not' getting involved. It applies to all ages.

---

The more we feel out of control as parents the more we tend to over-control our teens. Instead practice listening, encouraging, and coaching your teen through their struggles.

---

Instead of making it your goal to go out and find more information about parenting, try to do the simple things that you already know how to do and maybe just haven't applied.

---

Ask your teen for help. The things that might seem boring to you might energize them. Give them a chance to show you that they can make decisions and can handle adult tasks.

---

When your child is a pre-teen, you need to be there to protect and shelter, but the teenage years are different. Struggles and confusion are the building blocks for the future.

---

Try not to push your child into rapidly more mature roles. Let children be children - they need to work through the stages of development in order to gain the fullest benefits.

---

If you are losing perspective,

disclose your struggle with a trusted friend. Listen to more voices than your own when making an evaluation of how to move forward with your teen.

---

Many of the current leaders in America experienced war in their youth. Seeing struggle strengthened their generation. Why are we afraid of letting our kids experience hardship.

---

The hardest thing for anyone to do is say, I am sorry. Lead your family with this bold and courageous practice. It will heal many wounds and draw your family closer.

---

Teens have a sixth sense for the

weakness of their parents. If you demonstrate a willingness to compromise, back down, or retreat, you will bring out even more audacious behavior.

---

Anger is the best short-term method of gaining control within the home, but the technique with the least long term success. Do not burn relational bridges for momentary control.

---

Not only are parents stressed but kids are too. Kids often carry the anxiety and chaos of the home with them. Simplify your life and watch the hostility leave their lives as well.

---

Highlight the strengths of your

teen and let them know that you see them as an example for others. You'll set the bar high, and they will be motivated to live up to their reputations.

---

Mark significant moments in your child's life. These celebrations will remind us of our lasting connection and give perspective to the momentary difficulties that we might be facing.

---

The character you show as a parent is like a window into your life. Your teens can look into them and see what you really believe. Then they will decide whether to follow you or not.

---

Teens are often more bold verbally than they are internally. Do not match your teen's level of verbal aggression with anger. Teens really do not intend to be as hostile as they sound.

---

It is important to discuss decisions with your teen but be careful not to place your child's will above your own. Consider your own needs and feelings before consulting with your child.

---

When we as parents believe that everything we say or do is of critical importance to the psychological makeup of our child, we become paralyzed in fear and doubt our own wisdom as adults.

---

*It is critical for you to determine if you are the kind of parent that tends to over-control or to over-indulge. Controllers make all the decisions and those that indulge do not make any.*

---

*It is tempting to be near-sighted as we raise our children into teenagers. Be a parent that sees* far away. Keep the big picture in mind even when your child gets focused on small battles.

---

Parenting will always be an adventure, it isn't easy, and the process of parenting might change you more than you expect. Accept the challenge in order to prepare for the next phase of life.

---

*Anger is not the problem in most relationships. It is the inability to use anger as a healthy warning signal that something in your relationship needs work. Figure it out and then do the work.*

---

*It can be hard not to know what your teen is thinking or feeling. But* conducting rapid fire questioning or reading their private correspondence will only lead to greater distancing on their part.

---

Touch is a powerful weapon against anger for both you and your teen. Reach out and pat them on the back, hold their hand, share a hug. Let your presence speak louder than the aggressive language.

---

Children are too young to have a larger perspective. Do not get trapped in debates when they are focused on meeting their immediate desires. Widen the discussion with thought provoking questions.

---

Do not listen to the menacing voice

that sometimes whispers to our core, Close your heart. They do not deserve your love. He hates you. Do not let her hurt you again. Let him/her go.

---

As parents we often feel a need to control the decisions our child makes because we do not trust them to live within limits. This usually backfires into anger, rebellion, and emotional withdrawal.

---

Check your desire for power, dominance, and superiority. We often take our insecurities from work home with us and express disappointment with our kids as a way to feel morally superior to someone.

---

Anxiety is a by-product of increased access to information. Counteract this heightened awareness through limiting your own careless discussion of stressful situations in front of your young children.

---

Maybe we should stop lying to our kids. They deserve to learn the truth about their behaviors and how they effect us and others. Allow them to experience the natural consequences of their behavior.

---

As parents we can do many things to help shape and guide the experiences and decisions of our kids, but in the end your behavior as a parent does not completely determine the outcome of their lives.

*It is OK to let other adults help you parent even when you do not completely agree with their approach to life. Teens need to watch other approaches in action in order to value Mom and Dad is insight.*

How might you be trying to fix your parents' mistakes now as parents yourself? While some things might need improvement, we often over-reach and swing too far in the opposite direction. Find balance.

---

It is okay to let other adults help you parent even when you do not completely agree with their approach to life. Teens need to watch other approaches in action in order to value Mom and Dad's insight.

---

There is a lot of competition for our parent-child relationship. Maintain your parental satisfaction by not introducing competitive forces early in life like television, computer games, and cell phones.

---

Life is always full of change: change in health, change in finances, change in location and change in family dynamics. You cannot hold back change. Try to enjoy the new experiences change will bring you.

---

Battles with your teen often fall

into two categories: ethical/respect issues and personal preferences. Be willing to lose the personal preference battles in exchange for the more lasting ethical concerns.

---

Practice concealing your facial expressions. Teens are less able to project blame when your exterior is unreadable and flat. Sometimes any hint of a response can elicit the full emotion of their guilt.

---

If you think doing things yourself is easier because it avoids a battle with your teen, remember that the number one goal of every teen is to avoid work. Do not let their initial push back discourage you.

---

Do not allow your teens to miss opportunities to learn lessons from pain and failure. If they are forced to learn hard lessons later in life as adults, it is usually accompanied by more severe consequences.

---

Children without limits are insecure and afraid, and not able to verbalize these emotions. So they act out with misbehavior trying to force the authority in their lives to set a standard as a line of protection.

---

The world might feel more dangerous and competitive than the carefree times of your own youth... but it isn't.  Parent with confidence and watch your kids embrace the challenges in life rather than shrink in fear.

---

Always make sure you have 1-on-1 time with your child, especially if there are more kids on the way. It will create a memory and give them the extra attention you may not have time for after your new kids are born.

---

*The family unit is such a dynamic, interacting machine. Emotions come and go as they're stirred up in relationships. As you work through issues with your kids, do not hold onto the anger once the issues are resolved.*

---

*Being a parent is like being the CEO of a small company. Your kids* rely on you to inspire and stimulate them. Take time to learn what motivates them. Be optimistic; no one is going to follow a pessimistic leader.

---

Dependency on God and healthy dependency on others is invaluable during difficult times. We are not meant to have all the answers and to do it all on our own. Reach-out, receive the comfort that others can provide.

---

Most kids are looking for leadership in their lives. They will follow whomever demonstrates initiative. Are you sitting on the sidelines of parenthood? Kids want and need someone with integrity and self-motivation.

---

Don't listen to the menacing voice that sometimes whispers to our core, Close your heart. They don't deserve your love. He hates you. Don't let her hurt you again. Let him/her go.

---

Take time today to get to know your teen. Check in with them all the time. You can't lead someone you don't know. Teens are always changing and if you want to help them develop, you need to know who they are.

---

Think about what you are going to say to your teen before you say it. This works well with spouses too. Most communication is charged with history. Appreciate your influence and try to temper it with humility and understanding.

---

Trying to get leverage with our teens' lives often leads us to do crazy things as parents. We can become very manipulative and threatening. The closeness we desire will be eroded because the child feels inadequate or unacceptable.

Don't be a skunk. When a skunk is angry it sprays the thing it is angry at but everybody else has to smell it. Protect your kids from the stink by showing respect to your partner and working out your issues with respect and honor.

Do not be a skunk. When a skunk is angry it sprays the thing it's angry at but everybody else has to smell it. Protect your kids from the stink by showing respect to your partner and working out your issues with respect and honor.

---

Pushing kids into adult-like behaviors is like taking all of their exams for them in school and then being surprised that they fail in college. Let them struggle through each developmental stage so that their learning is deep and real.

---

If your 2 or 3 year old is having a tantrum and you have found that nothing works, put the child in a nice warm bubble bath. It is soothing, calming, and it makes them feel like they are back in the womb. I promise, it works every time!

---

Kids no longer look to iconic positions like presidents for leadership. When asked, kids generally choose a teacher, coach, or parent as the most inspirational leader in their lives. Are you the kind of leader that YOU would want to follow?

---

We all hate to be told what to do. Instead, ask your teen in a way that will make them feel as if they came up with the idea. Please do it this way turns into Do you think it's a good idea if we do it this way?

---

Are you so eager to be loved and

accepted by your kids that you will endure mistreatment? When you fix things for your kids in an attempt to win favor, it ends up hurting you and they never learn responsibility or respect for your rules.

---

Watch for open windows of communication with your teen. They do not come along often so do not let them slide by because you are too busy or afraid of their response. Start slowly like you're trying to feed a wild animal. You do not want to startle them.

---

Adding a 'call to action' is a standard sales technique and could be very helpful in parenting. Sometimes we never actually ask our kids to do specific things but are disappointed when they fail to live up to expectations. Be clear and make direct calls to action.

---

When our child is less than what we expect, we blame them. Why? Because if someone else is the source of the problem, then we have no responsibility to fix the problem and our anger is justified. Use your frustration as motivation to get involved and resolve the problem.

---

It is easy to lapse into using bribery to get jobs done or to avoid a tantrum (even from a teen). Reset expectations immediately if your child is not willingly contributing to family tasks like loading the dishwasher, cleaning up after themselves, or emptying the trash.

Progress is happening even when I can't see it. Embrace the absolute necessity for your child to make mistakes in order to grow. Every unwise choice is an opportunity, not a failure. It may be one more step toward your child growing tired of his current lifestyle.

*Helping your child reach adulthood is like sending a rocket into space. There is lots of smoke and fire, but in the end hitting the target relies on the proper direction from the beginning. Give your young child the rules, boundaries and support that they need to make the journey.*

---

*Hostility between parents often has*

a way of trickling down to the kids, whether or not they witness it directly. Kids will often try to punish parents if they perceive unfair treatment to have occurred between parents. It is critical to create a culture in which respect is valued.

---

Being well rounded should not be the goal. Striving for balance can force your teen to waste valuable time and energy and will usually end in arguments. Instead help them build on strengths and core competencies. Success in areas of natural strengths will lead them to try other more difficult areas in time.

---

Most of the famous leaders of today were risk-takers as teens.

They were willing to cut against the grain.? They were often oppositional during their adolescent years because they were forming the confidence and spunk that, when molded and crafted correctly, helped them to be productive and effective leaders as adults.

---

Remind yourself that it is the simple things in life that are the most helpful for growth. With a plethora of information and advice at our fingertips we tend to feel that there is some secret knowledge out there. Do not believe the lie that if we could just obtain that piece of information it would finally be the answer to our hopelessness, frustration, depression, or anger.

---

Give recognition and small rewards.

Internal family competition and challenges can be fun and highly motivating. Inviting your teen to participate in a 5K run, read a book, or go for a walk once a week to earn a tangible reward might give them the nudge in the right direction. Don't break the bank, but the reward of dinner out or a movie can motivate your teen while also creating memorable family time.

www.ingramcontent.com/pod-product-compliance
Lightning Source LLC
Chambersburg PA
CBHW051252250726
48656CB00004B/1251
* 9 7 9 8 3 2 0 0 8 8 5 6 3 *